ONLINE GAMING
SAFETY AND PRIVACY

JENNIFER CULP

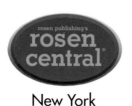

rosen publishing's
rosen central®

New York

Published in 2014 by The Rosen Publishing Group, Inc.
29 East 21st Street, New York, NY 10010

Library of Congress Cataloging-in-Publication Data

Culp, Jennifer.
Online gaming safety and privacy/Jennifer Culp. — 1st ed. —
New York: Rosen, © 2014
         p. cm. — (21st century safety and privacy)
Includes bibliographical references and index.
ISBN: 978-1-4488-9570-0 (Library Binding)
ISBN: 978-1-4488-9584-7 (Paperback)
ISBN: 978-1-4488-9585-4 (6-pack)
1. Internet games—Juvenile literature. 2. Internet and children—
Juvenile literature. 3. Internet—Security measures—Juvenile literature.
4. Internet—Safety measures—Juvenile literature. 5. Privacy, Right of—
Juvenile literature. I. Title.
GV1469.15 .C85 2014
794.8

Manufactured in the United States of America

CPSIA Compliance Information: Batch #S13YA: For further information, contact Rosen Publishing, New York, New York,
at 1-800-237-9932.

CONTENTS

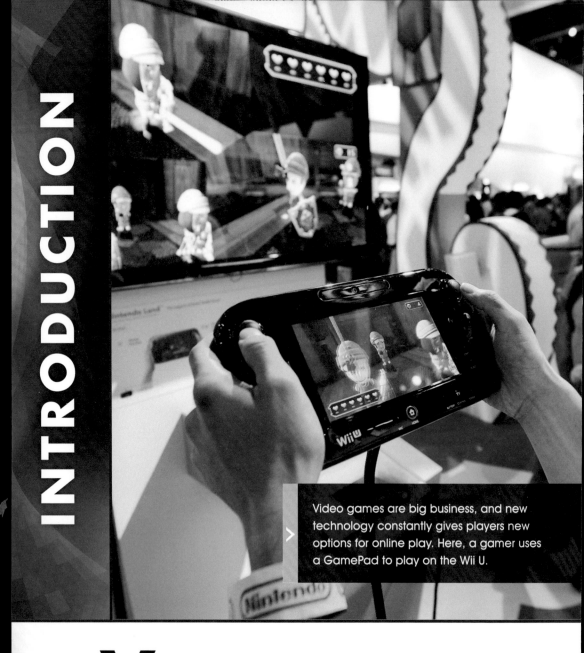

INTRODUCTION

Video games are big business, and new
technology constantly gives players new
options for online play. Here, a gamer uses
a GamePad to play on the Wii U.

Video games are becoming increasingly popular.
A recent study from the Pew Internet & American
Life Project revealed that 97 percent of teens ages twelve
to seventeen play games on a computer, game console,

portable handheld device, or phone. Many teens connect with others to play games online, and there has never been a greater variety of games with online play options. Online gaming services such as Xbox Live, PlayStation Network, and Nintendo Wi-Fi Connection allow players to access the Internet through their game consoles. Others play massively multiplayer online role-playing games, such as *World of Warcraft*, on a computer. Handheld gaming devices such as the Nintendo DSi allow players to compare scores, send messages, and even share photos with one another. Many people who don't even think of themselves as typical "gamers" spend time playing social games such as *FarmVille* or *Words with Friends*, made available online through Facebook. A three-year study of thirteen- to sixteen-year-olds conducted by researchers from Brunel University even showed that online gaming may in fact be beneficial for teenagers, giving opportunities for exploration and social interaction that may not be available in "real life."

Despite all of its positive aspects, there are very real dangers associated with playing online. It's important to be aware of these problems so that you can avoid them and have fun playing online safely.

CHAPTER ONE

WHAT'S THE DANGER?

Online gaming is fun, but it can potentially lead to trouble. Being aware of the possible dangers associated with playing on the Internet can help you avoid pitfalls and play in safety.

It's Just a Game

When you sit down and turn on your Xbox or other gaming system, it can feel like you're escaping into another world. You get to explore new landscapes and tackle creative challenges. When you lose a turn or even get a "Game Over" screen, it's no big deal; you can just reload and try again, all from the comfort of your own couch. Nothing can really hurt you in a game, right?

Wrong. Like the name says, online gaming takes place online—over the Internet. Even though you might connect to the Internet through a game console instead of a computer to play, you still face the same risks commonly associated

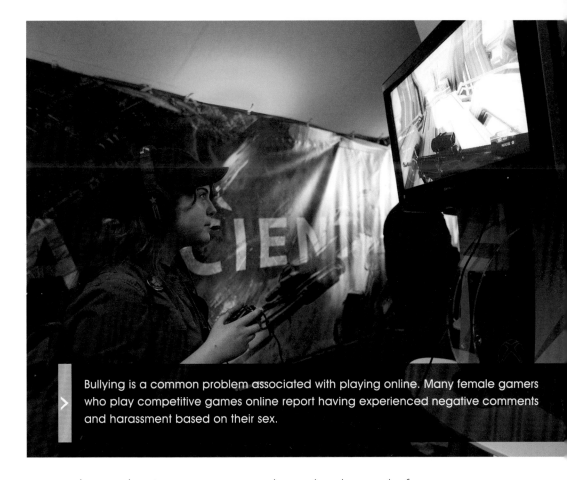

> Bullying is a common problem associated with playing online. Many female gamers who play competitive games online report having experienced negative comments and harassment based on their sex.

with regular Internet use, such as hacking, theft, privacy violation, and bullying. You're still playing a game, but the minute you connect to the Internet, you become vulnerable to its dangers—even if you're playing by yourself. In online multiplayer games, unfortunately, not everyone you encounter may have your best interests in mind.

Hackers

Hacking is a problem across many platforms, not just computers. In most cases, hackers want access to players' gaming accounts in order to purchase game content for themselves or to steal players' credit card information in order to buy things unrelated to the game. Some hackers, or "jackers," as some who don't use traditional hacking methods to break into others' accounts call themselves, aren't even interested in financial gain. They might want to steal an account because of its rightful owner's impressive playing record or cool username.

Bullying and Harassment

Other online attacks are intended to cause emotional damage. Bullying is unfortunately common in online gaming and can take a wide variety of forms, from harassing messages, lewd or threatening "chat," or repeated efforts to foil a specific player's efforts in the game. Mean-spirited conversation during play and cruel messages are so prevalent that there are Web sites dedicated to showing particularly bad examples and exposing the screen names of the gamers responsible. Some people bully indiscriminately, just trying to ruin everyone's good time instead of focusing on a particular target. This concerted effort toward mayhem and destruction is known as "griefing." Griefers, as those who engage in this behavior are known, enjoy irritating other players and prevent them from playing a game normally. Some griefers might target a specific player or players, stalking their victims across different games and even online gaming services in order to ruin their gameplay

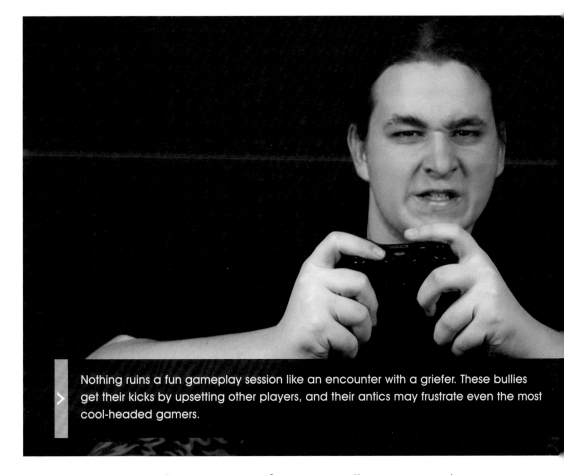

> Nothing ruins a fun gameplay session like an encounter with a griefer. These bullies get their kicks by upsetting other players, and their antics may frustrate even the most cool-headed gamers.

experiences. The term "griefing" actually originated in online gaming, and it has since come to include any form of purposefully annoying or hurtful behavior aimed at others on the Internet.

Less common but perhaps most chilling, sexual predation is also a danger to young players in online gaming. These criminals often disguise themselves as fellow underage peers in order to gain a young gamer's trust before seeking to solicit inappropriate pictures or meet in person for ill purposes.

> BULLYING IN ONLINE GAMING

Bullying is extremely prevalent in online gaming. Anonymity and the heightened emotions caused by competition can make online games a breeding ground for bad behavior. A bully may employ many tactics to hurt another player, including:

- Profanity, lewd language, and name-calling over voice chat or in written messages
- Targeting a specific player for harm in a manner not intended by the game's creators
- Intentional "friendly fire" or other actions to frustrate a teammate's progress, such as stealing a quest item or blocking someone from leaving an area
- Spamming a chat channel to interrupt other players' communication
- Written or verbal threats
- Attempting to impersonate a player to damage his or her reputation with other players

If someone is bullying you, most online gaming services offer a way to block contact with the offender and report the bad behavior, which may result in punishment such as suspension or even being banned from the service. Additionally, you should not hesitate to take action if you see a friend engage in these activities.

Why Should This Stuff Matter to Me?

All of those things are terrible, you might think, but they'll never happen to me. They happen only to a few people, right? Or they happen only to irresponsible people who play violent, mature-rated games.

Wrong.

In autumn 2011, some users of Xbox Live noticed that their accounts had been used to play *FIFA 12*, a soccer simulation game, and that unauthorized purchases of downloadable content on Xbox Live had been made with their credit cards. Some of the victims lost even more money as the hackers were able to make very expensive purchases through the stolen Xbox Live members' linked PayPal accounts. Twenty-three-year-old Susan Taylor had never played *FIFA 12* when her Xbox Live account was hacked in early 2012. Although she had taken reasonable safety precautions and her Xbox Live and PayPal accounts did not share usernames or passwords, the two services were linked via her Xbox system. Susan was not the victim of a "phishing" scam, in which a hacker tricks a player into revealing account log-in information, but merely unlucky. She went on to found the Web site Hacked on Xbox in order to share her story, help others who have been hacked, and spread information about how to prevent or combat Xbox Live account hijacking. The site features stories from some of the thousands of

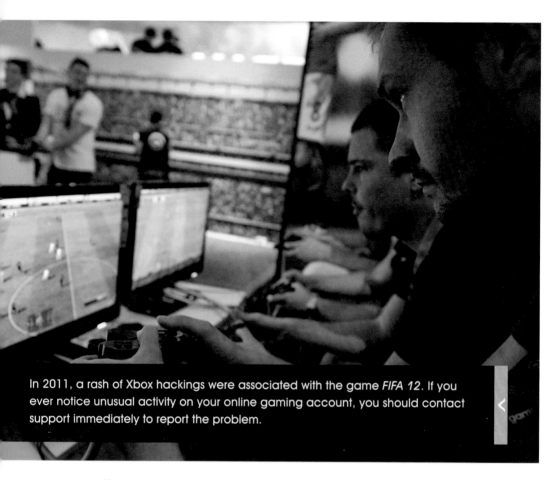

In 2011, a rash of Xbox hackings were associated with the game *FIFA 12*. If you ever notice unusual activity on your online gaming account, you should contact support immediately to report the problem.

different people who are hacked each year. This kind of account hijacking could easily happen to a friend or a family member, or it could even happen to you.

In one of the largest data breaches in history, the PlayStation Network (PSN) was hacked in April 2011, providing the culprits with access to all PlayStation Network account information and passwords for every one of the more than seventy million users of PSN. Sony, the company that owns PlayStation, was forced to shut down the entire online service in order to investigate the scope of the break-in and set it right. You probably know people who were affected by this hack. If you had a PlayStation Network account in 2011, your information was compromised in this attack.

Bullying in online gaming is tragically widespread. Data from the Pew Internet & American Life Project implies that nearly everyone who plays online will at least witness, if not personally experience, offensive or antisocial behavior. Bullying and griefing are widespread across all social gaming platforms. They are so widespread, in fact, that it's difficult to boil down to a few printable examples. The line between griefing and bullying is blurry. A griefer may set out to cause mayhem impartially but decide to target a specific player or players for harassment. Bullies might set out to hurt someone they know from real life in the virtual world or may begin to bully a stranger who beat them at a game. Some instances of bullying are relatively harmless and some incredibly damaging and hurtful, but none whatsoever are acceptable.

MYTHS AND FACTS

Myth: Girls don't play online video games.

Fact: The Entertainment Software Association's 2012 report on sales, demographic, and usage data revealed that the percentage of total female gamers had risen to 47 percent, an increase from the 2011 report.

Myth: Playing online games is just a waste of time.

Fact: Game designer, researcher, and author Jane McGonigal's 2011 book *Reality Is Broken: Why Games Make Us Better and How They Can Change the World* compiles the results of numerous scientific studies to conclude that overall, people who spend time playing online games tend to be happier, more productive, more skilled at problem solving, and more enthusiastic about interacting with other people than those who do not engage in online gaming.

Myth: All online games are violent, multiplayer shooting games.

Fact: There are a huge number of different online games for all ages, ranging from sports and racing games on the Xbox 360, PlayStation 3, and Wii to fighting games on a desktop computer to handheld console titles such as *Pokémon* to social media games that are played on Facebook.

PERSONAL INFORMATION AND THE IMPORTANCE OF PRIVACY

As we've established, there are dangers associated with online gaming. The good news is that a little caution and common sense can go a long way toward keeping you safe while playing.

Preventing Danger by Protecting Privacy

Imagine that you're Link in a *Legend of Zelda* game. When you prepare to enter the final dungeon and tackle the evil tyrant Ganondorf, you're not going to leave your Master Sword behind. If you're smart, you'll take the time to stock up on extra precautions, like a spare health potion that gives you an extra life, which will give you a better chance at defeating the final boss and winning the game.

When you set out to play on a new online platform, you're a hero starting out on your own epic quest. Don't leave yourself vulnerable to enemies by neglecting

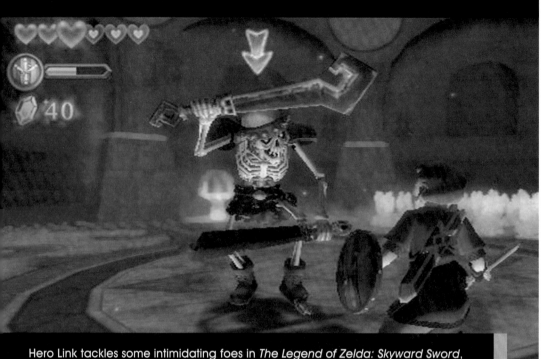

Hero Link tackles some intimidating foes in *The Legend of Zelda: Skyward Sword*, but stays safe by keeping his shield in good condition. Your shield against online threats is common sense and caution.

your armor. Your most valuable possession in the online world is your personal information, and your strongest shield is privacy. This shield gets weaker and weaker if it gets "cracked" by you sharing your information with others. The best strategy to keep it strong and keep yourself safe is simple: *keep private information to yourself.*

Phishing

"Phishing" is a tactic hackers use to steal passwords, user-names, and credit card information by pretending to be a trustworthy person or organization online. Phishing plagues all forms of online communication, including gaming. By befriending and learning some details about a gamer's life, a hacker or account hijacker can go on to break into the victim's online gaming profile, hack into e-mail or social media accounts, impersonate the gamer, or even access bank information to steal money. In the online world, most of your information is linked up in some way. If a hacker gets some of your information in one online arena, your entire online presence is vulnerable. Don't hand out information to someone who might use it to steal from you or your family.

Fortunately, it's easy to keep your private information private. Do you know another gamer in real life? If not, then don't tell him or her your name, age, or gender. No one else in your online match needs to know where you live, and they *certainly* don't need to know your mother's maiden name. While chatting in-game or messaging over Xbox Live or PlayStation Network, keep conversation limited to game topics only. If someone you don't know asks for details about your offline life, don't answer. If the person continues to ask, you'll know that he or she shouldn't be trusted.

If someone does put a crack in your privacy shield, move quickly to patch it up. Change the password for your online gaming account, e-mail, and social media accounts, and be careful to keep your lips zipped in the future. Remember: if it's not related to the game you're playing, it's not an appropriate topic for discussion with another player.

Deceitful individual hackers aren't the only threats to your online gaming armor. Sometimes the company that makes the game itself is after your information. User agreements for individual games are full of important stuff. They are usually long and written in confusing legal terms, and it's tempting to skip right past and play your new game immediately. If you do that, however, you'll never know exactly what info you agreed to give the company when you started playing the game. All games collect

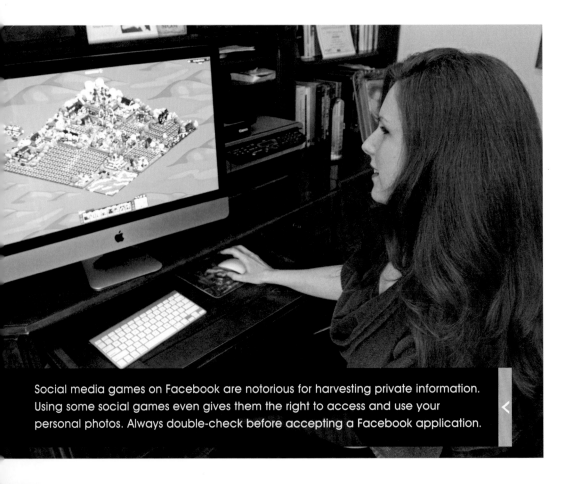

Social media games on Facebook are notorious for harvesting private information. Using some social games even gives them the right to access and use your personal photos. Always double-check before accepting a Facebook application.

some demographic information to improve their games and better market them in the future. That's not a terribly big deal. But some games may share your information with third parties, and you should know where your info is going before clicking the "OK" button. When you scan a user agreement, pay attention to sections that detail what kind of information the game will collect about you and whether or not that information will be shared with other companies, or third parties. This is particularly important when signing up for social media games such as *FarmVille*, *Words with Friends*, or *Draw Something*. Some social media games require access not only to your Facebook account and password, for instance, but your friends list, photos, and other applications as well. Always make sure you know what you're signing up for. If you're giving a gaming company a higher value in information than you're receiving in enjoyment from playing the game, you're getting ripped off.

Finally, make sure you're familiar with your online gaming platform so that you can ensure you're as well-protected as possible. Services such as Xbox Live and PlayStation Network update their layouts from time to time (and Facebook, well, it's constantly changing). Sit down with an adult and explore all of your account options. You should always know what information is contained in your public profile. Anonymous username and picture, gamer score, achievements, and trophies you've earned by completing game objectives are fine. But if a public profile reveals any

> CODENAME: SAFE GAMER

Most online gaming services require you to create a username or gamertag, a pseudonym that identifies you to other players. It can be tempting to choose a username that reflects you and your interests, but doing so can reveal information that is best kept private.

Think of your gamertag as your secret identity. Try to make your name as incognito as possible. Instead of basing your username on your real name or an activity you enjoy, pick some random words that you like and string them out together. Don't include your birth date in your username. Keep your gender under wraps, too.

Likewise, it's natural to want to make your avatar in a game or online gaming profile look like you, but it's best to resist the urge. Instead of making a self—portrait out of your Mii or Xbox Live avatar, make it the face of your secret gaming identity. In online games that require you to make a character, think of how the character would look and act instead of yourself. What would he or she be like? Would your character have blue skin? Spiky orange hair? Have fun with it! Keeping a secret identity online lets you experiment with things that aren't possible in real life *and* keeps the real you safer.

personal info about you—real name, age, gender, location, etc.—you need to figure out how to remove it. You want to make sure that any wireless Internet connection you use to game is password protected and that any sharing service on your playable handheld console is deactivated unless you're in a safe location. Any privacy setting options should always be set to limit or prevent any visibility to strangers.

Keeping your online gaming armor polished by choosing optimal settings on your online gaming account or accounts takes time and effort. Technology is always changing, and keeping your public information as tight as possible requires near constant maintenance. It's simple enough to get into a routine of checking out any changes to your online gaming accounts and making sure they're in good order, though. This small investment of time and discipline pays off big time in protecting your privacy.

But What About Friends?

Just as you shouldn't share real-life information with online gaming acquaintances, another important step to protecting your privacy is keeping personal gaming information secret from your real-life friends. This doesn't mean that your friends shouldn't know your Xbox gamertag or that it should be a secret that you play *Madden NFL 13*. In that case, how would they play with you? In this case, private information is information that gives access to your account or allows someone to impersonate you. You should never, *ever* let a friend have access to your password: not your best friend, not your boyfriend, not your girlfriend. Nor should you let any of your friends play a game on one of your accounts if you're not there to supervise.

"What's the big deal if my friend has my password?" you might wonder. Sharing an account might initially seem like a good idea. It's not. You've probably seen someone you know get "hacked" on Facebook or Twitter, when they've left their account open and someone else posts a joke status on the account. That can happen in

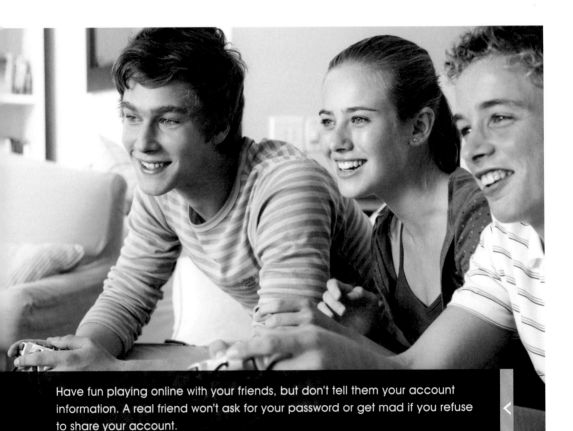

Have fun playing online with your friends, but don't tell them your account information. A real friend won't ask for your password or get mad if you refuse to share your account.

online gaming accounts, too. If someone else has access to your gaming account, that person can use it for more than just playing games. Someone could change your status or picture, or send messages to others. If someone behaves badly while playing a game, it won't damage his or her own reputation, but it could do irreparable damage to yours. If someone uses your account to grief or troll other players, you could get suspended or banned from playing your own game. A friend with access to your password could even log in to your account, change your password to something you don't know, and lock you out of your own account. Online gaming is supposed to be fun, but if you give your friends license to impersonate you, it can turn into a social battlefield. Play games with your friends. Don't give them your password. Real friends respect boundaries, and real friends help you protect your privacy. Someone who truly cares about you won't continue to press you to divulge your password after you've said no.

Unblockable Attacks

While playing a game, you sometimes come up against an unblockable attack. As anyone who's been knocked out of first place by a blue shell in *Mario Kart* knows, unblockable attacks are really frustrating. There's nothing you can do to prevent the initial damage, but with some recuperative effort and luck, you might be able to catch back up and win the race.

Despite the best privacy protection practices, people can fall victim to plain bad luck. An interview with a teenage Xbox hacker on the gaming Web site Kotaku details the practice of "social engineering"—basically, phishing for information from customer service representatives, rather than individual gamers. In these cases, a hacker impersonates a gamer and convinces a customer service representative to reset the password for an account, allowing the hacker to access the account and lock its owner out. In spite of the most excellent privacy protection, it can still be possible for a hacker with ill intent to glean enough basic information (such as a username and e-mail address) to fool a customer service representative into giving up access to the account.

This is basically an unblockable attack. The stolen information wasn't provided by the victim, and there's little he or she could have done to prevent it. In this case, the important thing is to act to fix the problem quickly. Fifteen-year-old "Sean B" shared his story of resolving a similar problem on the Web site Hacked on Xbox. When Sean's brother tried to log on to their shared account and found that the password had been changed, Sean knew something was wrong. He immediately called Microsoft, the company that owns Xbox, to report the issue. After verifying that Sean was the account holder, a Microsoft representative was able to help him transfer his information to a new account. Sean had used his grandmother's credit card to make purchases on Xbox Live, so he informed his family and the Microsoft representative about possible fraudulent charges made with the card. Microsoft refunded the money that the hacker had stolen from Sean's grandmother, which his family confirmed by checking with the credit card company. In this unfortunate situation, Sean achieved a nearly ideal resolution by quickly noticing the problem, immediately calling a customer service representative for help, keeping his family informed and involved in the process, and double-checking the outcome with the game company and credit card company. In a similar situation, responding quickly and keeping detailed track of the events is the best thing you can do.

It's advisable to keep up with news about your gaming service of choice. When the entire PlayStation Network was hacked in 2011, obviously no one individual PSN user could have prevented this attack on his or her own personal account. Sony, the company that owns PSN, was responsible for fixing the breach of information, but it was up to individual gamers to change their passwords for not only their PSN accounts but all of their online accounts as well.

CHAPTER THREE

WHAT'S SAFE AND WHAT'S NOT?

There is a huge variety of online games and different platforms to play on, and an even bigger variety of people who play all of them. It can be overwhelming to contemplate safety concerns when you're faced with so many choices. Keeping a few simple guidelines in mind can help you pick the right games and stay safe while playing.

Do Your Research

Knowing *what* you're playing helps keep you safe *while* you're playing. Learning about the online gaming service you use to play, such as Xbox Live, PlayStation Network, and Nintendo Wi-Fi Connection, is important. Checking user agreements before playing specific games lets you know what kind of information a game collects and how that information might be used in future research and marketing. Before that, though, it's important to have some understanding of the game's content.

The Entertainment Software Rating Board (ESRB) gives every game marketed in the United States and Canada a rating to indicate appropriateness for different audiences, similar to movie ratings. Retailers may not sell "mature" M-rated games to anyone under the age of seventeen. T-rated "teen" games may have some inappropriate content for kids under the age of thirteen, but they may be purchased with parental permission. E-rated games are suitable for all audiences. The ESRB cannot control—and

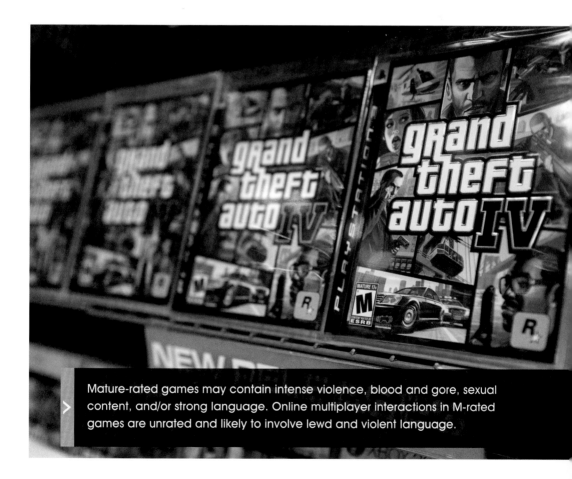

Mature-rated games may contain intense violence, blood and gore, sexual content, and/or strong language. Online multiplayer interactions in M-rated games are unrated and likely to involve lewd and violent language.

therefore does not rate—online interactions, but these ratings can still serve as a pretty good indicator of what kind of communication you can expect while playing a multiplayer game online. A T-rated shooter game may attract heightened competitiveness and more trash talking during play than an E-rated puzzle game. Many of the most egregious examples of lewd language and harassment take place in the multiplayer modes of M-rated games that contain violence and adult content. This doesn't always hold true, but it is an easy rule of thumb when first evaluating a game: the higher the ESRB rating, the worse most gamers will behave in multiplayer arenas.

It's wise to ask questions about a game you're interested in before buying. Many games offer online play, but each one is different. Can you choose whom to play with online and join up with friends, or does the game automatically place you in matches with strangers? The salesperson at a video game store or some basic Internet research should be able to let you know if a game is a good match for your needs. Don't be afraid to ask. Additionally, some games are more prone to griefing or hacking than others. A knowledgeable sales associate should be able to advise you on whether a certain game or franchise has been known to be associated with any specific dangers.

Playing with Strangers

Some online games are single-player. There are downloadable classic games like *Frogger* or games like

Angry Birds, which can be played on a Web browser or smartphone. In social games, like *ChefVille*, you help friends by giving them recipe ingredients or dining in their restaurants, but you don't actually interact with them in real time. These are all online games, but when most people talk about gaming online, they mean playing in online multiplayer matches with and against other people. A big part of the allure of online gaming is testing your skills against other living, breathing human beings

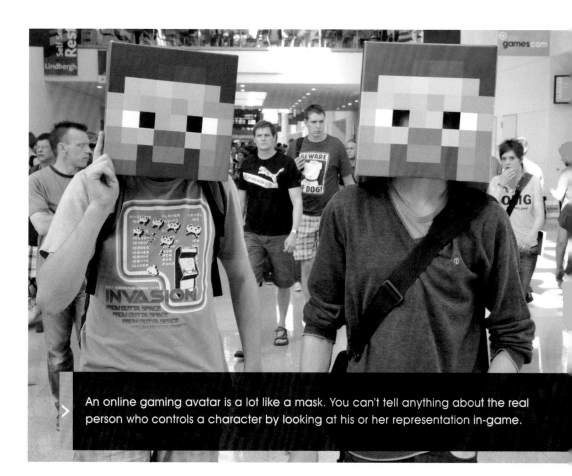

An online gaming avatar is a lot like a mask. You can't tell anything about the real person who controls a character by looking at his or her representation in-game.

around the world, rather than simply playing against a computer.

Playing online with others can be a lot of fun. After countless hours of playing with the same people, it can feel like you really know them. Sometimes people do become good friends after meeting anonymously online. It's important to remember, however, that the people you meet in-game are not the real, living people controlling the characters.

Someone who acts clingy or wants to be your BFF without any contact outside of Xbox Live or PlayStation Network is decidedly not someone you can trust. Why is this person using gameplay as such an intense social outlet? Does he or she not have any friends or acquaintances in real life? In-game chat and messaging should focus around one thing: the game itself. That doesn't mean it can't be fun or that you can't joke, but non-game-related discussion can quickly turn fishy. Remember, the reason the various personalities behind the avatars have gathered together is to build an incredible castle in *Minecraft* or strategize against another cohort of players in *Team Fortress 2*. You should be suspicious of anyone who wants to discuss unrelated topics or who continually questions you about personal information, particularly if you've asked the person to stop.

It's very unlikely that a person who makes boastful claims during gameplay is exactly the person he or she claims to be. The person may want to live out an alternate reality as a cooler, more popular person than he or she is in real life or could have more sinister intentions. If someone seems

> CHOOSING AN
> ONLINE GAME

So you've decided you want to play an online game. Great! Here are some steps for acquiring a new game:

1. Decide why you want to play this particular game. Is it a popular new release? Is it a specific type of game (racing, sports, combat) that you want to play? Think about why you want to play this particular game before impulsively grabbing it.

2. Talk to your parents.
   Sit down with your parents or guardian to talk about the game. Tell them why you want it. They might not be impressed if you want it just because it's a hot new property all your friends covet, but if you are truly inter—ested in the game mechanics or plot, it might be a different story.

3. Research.
   With your parents or guardian, do some research on the game. Does it have an appropriate ESRB rating? What kind of online multiplayer options does it offer? Make sure the game will align with your expectations and your parents' requirements. If it passes the research test...

4. Buy the game!

5. Once you've bought a game, remember that you're not quite done yet.
   Before playing, check to see what kind of information about you it gathers and, more important, what kind of information it shares with others. Check to make sure your privacy settings are optimal and make sure you have a good understanding of how the game will match you up to play with strangers before beginning.

6. Enjoy!

nosy about you—the real you, not your game character—he or she is most likely up to no good. Someone who's lying online or flattering you in order to learn things about you is not a real friend. It may seem like a good idea to call out perpetrators of this behavior, to catch them in the act and ask them to own up to their shady behavior, but it's not. If people seem too good to be true, they probably are. Attempting to expose someone's deception could make the person feel angry or vengeful. Just cut off contact and move on. If someone's behavior strikes you as potentially dangerous, consider reporting the behavior to your online gaming service.

A big red flag of *very* suspicious behavior is any display of romantic interest from someone you know only from a game. No one falls in love solely through playing a game together without meeting or truly knowing one another. It's very rare for adults to strike up a romantic connection during online play. Someone who professes love or even interest in a date with an underage player is shady. In 2012, *ABC News* reported the story of thirteen-year-old Beth Robinson, who met twelve-year-old "Dylan" on Xbox Live while playing the M-rated game *Call of Duty*. Their relationship developed over hours of gameplay and messages, and eventually they made a plan for Beth to run away and meet Dylan in his home in Kentucky. Beth stole her brother's car and mother's debit card, and using tips from Dylan to conceal her identity, made it as far as Nashville, Tennessee, before being apprehended by police. After the police returned Beth home safely, her father agreed to allow her to meet up with Dylan under parental supervision. When the Robinson family searched for the address Dylan had given Beth, however, they couldn't locate it anywhere. Beth's age-appropriate love "Dylan" didn't exist.

Why did Beth decide to run away in the first place? "Dylan" had earned her trust. He was the mastermind behind her plan to run away, giving her ideas to hide herself from authorities by switching the license plate of her brother's car. Fortunately, Beth was apprehended before she met up with the person who talked her into running from her family, but her story could have ended very differently. In 2011, several news outlets, including the *Escapist*, reported on the case of Rachel Ann Hicks, a thirty-six-year-old mother of three from California who was charged with rape and child molestation after traveling to meet and seduce her thirteen-year-old "boyfriend" in Maryland. Over Xbox Live, she had convinced him that she was a younger woman by sending him romantic messages under a false identity. After the boy's family members alerted local authorities, it took no less than the FBI to track the woman down, as she had provided her victim with a false name and age.

Have fun playing with the people you meet while gaming online. Talk to them about the game, joke with them, have a good time. Always remember, though, that you don't really know them. If you get a bad feeling about

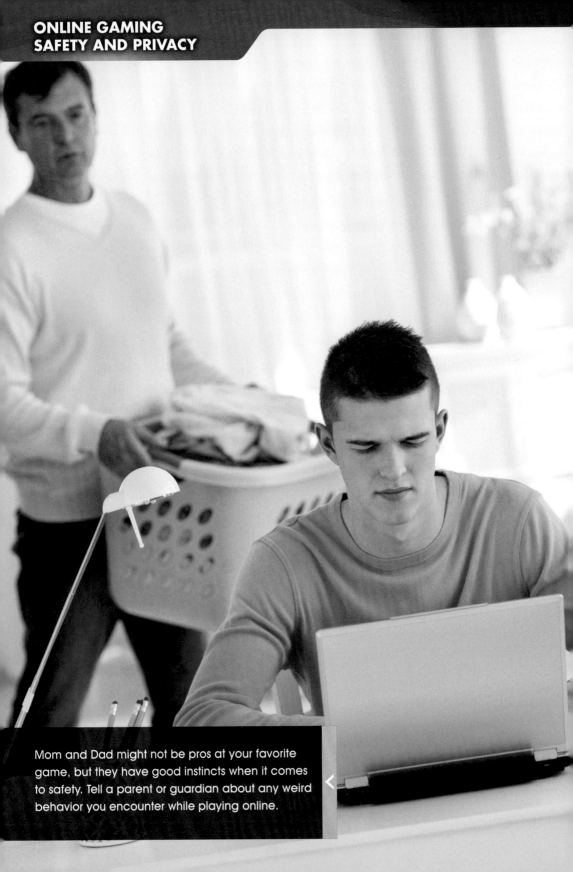

Mom and Dad might not be pros at your favorite game, but they have good instincts when it comes to safety. Tell a parent or guardian about any weird behavior you encounter while playing online.

another gamer, trust your instincts. If anyone says something suspicious to you or tries to pry information from you, tell an adult and report the behavior to your gaming service.

Sometimes it can be tempting to confide in online friends. Occasionally, when offline life is tough, someone you talk to online may even seem like a better friend than the people you know in real life. The "person" you know online is just make-believe, however, a character created by a real person. Never hand valuable information about yourself over to a fantasy. Don't put your trust in someone you don't really know. The real person behind the character you're playing with may be very different from the way he or she comes across as an online persona.

10 GREAT QUESTIONS

1 What's your favorite online game, and why?

2 What's your least favorite online game? How does it differ from your favorite?

3 What do you benefit from playing online multiplayer games?

4 Do you consider online gaming an important part of your social life? Why?

5 Has anyone ever said anything offensive to you while you were playing online? If so, how did you handle it?

6 What do you consider the most important safety concern in online gaming?

7 Do you have any suggestions for limiting exposure to bullies and griefers?

8 If you could design the perfect online game, what would it be like?

9 What was your favorite video game when you were my age? Did it have an interactive multiplayer option?

10 What current online game would you recommend for someone my age to play?

SOMETHING'S WRONG. WHAT SHOULD I DO?

CHAPTER FOUR

Despite the best preventative privacy practices, things occasionally go wrong. Don't panic! Problems can be fixed. Stay calm, identify the problem, and then take the right steps to resolve it.

Bullies and Griefers

Of all the potential dangers involved in playing online games, experiencing unpleasant behavior from others is by far the most common. According to the Pew Internet & American Life Project, 63 percent of teens who play games reported seeing or hearing "people being mean and overly aggressive while playing," and 49 percent reported seeing or hearing "people being hateful, racist, or sexist" while playing. Just about anyone who plays online multiplayer games regularly has at least one story about witnessing or directly experiencing lewdness, threats, or insults.

Many players have taken a turn at both roles in this situation. In a 2012 article published by the University of Michigan Journalism School, sixteen-year-old *Minecraft* player Andrew spoke about the problem of griefing in *Minecraft*. The object of *Minecraft* is to use blocks to build creations limited only by a person's imagination. A common objective of griefers in *Minecraft*, therefore, is to destroy hours of work laboriously accomplished by other gamers. Although Andrew spoke about playing the game on a protected server with friends in order to avoid such harassment, he admits to having griefed other players in the past.

If you experience harassment from a griefer or group of griefers, it is best not to respond, as this can escalate the behavior. Turning the game off and walking away for a while is often the best course of action. It's impossible to grief a player who isn't playing, and this can encourage griefers to leave you alone

Don't let griefers get to you. If you feel tempted to take revenge, shut the game down and take a break. Block them, report them, and move on.

long enough to block them on your online gaming service or set up preventative measures, such as restricting online play to your approved friends list or joining a protected server. It can be tempting to try to take revenge on a griefer and ruin his or her game in turn, but doing so can easily prompt the griefer to respond in kind. The best way to take vengeance on a griefer is to take advantage of your gaming service provider's report function. Game companies don't like griefing, as it hurts their players and drives them away from games. Nearly every online gaming service offers a way to report antisocial griefing or bullying activity to the company, which can then take action against the offender. Checking out the procedure for reporting bullies before you ever experience griefing is a good idea, but if you don't know how to report someone who turns up to ruin your good time, don't panic. Stay calm, make a note of the person's username, exit the game, and then look up how to report his or her actions.

Griefing is often broad and intended to cause as much mayhem and destruction to as many players as possible. Sometimes this type of bullying takes a more individually focused turn. A griefer may focus on a specific gamer and follow the person across platforms. In this case, remaining calm and attentive and continually reporting every offense to your game service provider or game moderators is the best way to respond. In extreme instances, bullied gamers have changed their own usernames in order to "start fresh" and avoid harassment. This is unadvisable unless

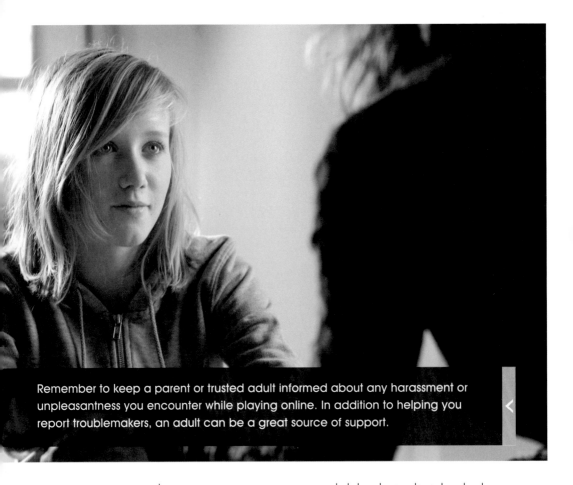

Remember to keep a parent or trusted adult informed about any harassment or unpleasantness you encounter while playing online. In addition to helping you report troublemakers, an adult can be a great source of support.

repeated attempts to report and block individuals have not succeeded in defusing the situation. Keep cooperating with game company representatives; they have a vested interest in protecting you and removing griefers from their servers.

In other circumstances, bullying can be even more personal. When friends or acquaintances turn to bullying, it can be difficult to avoid them because they may be able to track usernames easily among a friend group, talk their way onto protected servers run by friends, and even convince

> DON'T GIVE
> ANY GRIEF

Griefing holds a certain allure. There are well-liked videos of griefing exploits on YouTube. Friends might cheer you on in partaking in mean-spirited behavior. For a brief moment, hurting someone else can feel like a big thrill.

When it's not *your* game being ruined, griefing doesn't seem like a problem. As long as *you're* having a good time, who cares about other players? You don't even know them. Maybe your own friends think your griefing antics are funny. Why does it matter if some stranger gets angry, so long as you don't have to deal with the consequences?

There are, however, consequences to griefing. Gaming companies do not appreciate griefers who harass other players and interfere with a game's intended functioning. Xbox Live, PlayStation Network, MMORPGs such as *World of Warcraft*, and others level penalties on reported griefers, sometimes banning them outright from using the service. By griefing others, you risk losing the character you've devoted time to building in a game and even your entire online gaming account on a gaming service. It's not worth the risk.

friends that their actions are at best harmless or at worst funny. These bullies should be reported to gaming services just like any other griefer, but they should also be reported to parents or other trusted adults. Seek an adult's help to defuse this situation.

Always tell a parent or trusted adult about *any* hostile treatment you receive while playing online. Besides lending a sympathetic ear, adults have more resources at their disposal to deal with bullies and griefers. An adult with an objective viewpoint can often help you determine whether another player is dangerous and, if so, decide on the appropriate action to take.

Beyond Bullying

Although you should always inform a parent or trusted adult about any griefing or bullying you experience, you can resolve some minor situations yourself—*with* a parent's approval and guidance. A parent can help you block bullies from contacting you and report any harassment. If you notice anything strange that indicates your account may have been hacked or personal information stolen, however, it is imperative to inform an adult and let him or her take the necessary steps to solve the problem.

If you ever notice strange activity on any of your online gaming accounts, you should do two things: change your password (if possible) and tell a parent. You should also change the passwords of any accounts associated with your username, and your parent or guardian should change passwords and check bank accounts and any other financial accounts to see whether money has been stolen or used to make unauthorized purchases. Next, your parent or guardian should contact your online gaming service to

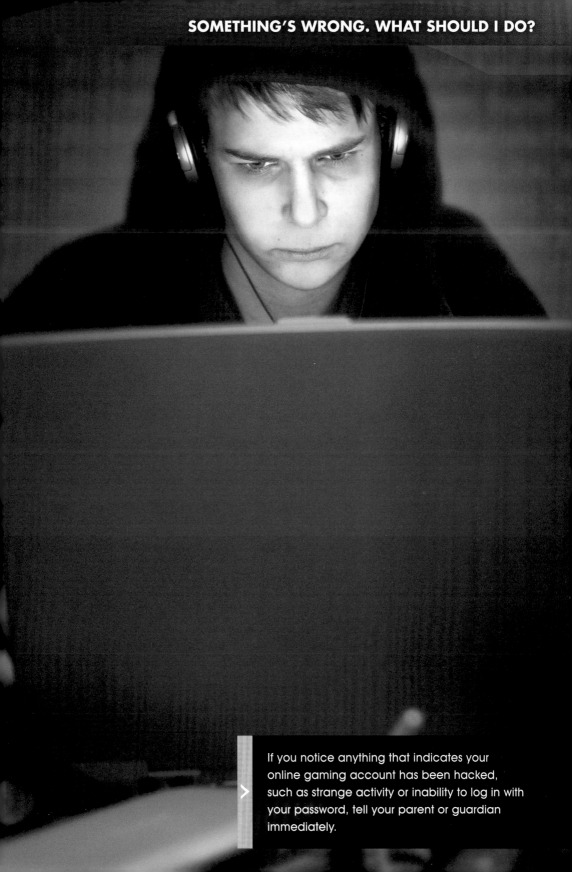

> If you notice anything that indicates your online gaming account has been hacked, such as strange activity or inability to log in with your password, tell your parent or guardian immediately.

report the hack. Following your gaming service representative's directives to rectify the situation and following up with any involved financial institutions are the only recourses in this case. In the case of any delay, your parent or guardian should be firm and persistent until the matter is sufficiently resolved. Everyone wants to see hackers and thieves brought to justice, but local law enforcement is very limited in this situation. A representative from the hacked gaming service may have advice on what sort of legal recourse, if any, your family should seek.

Finally, don't beat yourself up! An unblockable attack can happen to anyone, regardless of the best precautions. Stay calm, report the problem, and cooperate with the instructions of company representatives and authorities to ensure the best possible outcome.

PLAY IT SAFE WITH YOUR FRIENDS

Part of the fun of gaming is playing with your real-life friends. Playing online with strangers can be even more fun with a friend by your side, and everyone has a better time when their peers stay safe.

Friends Defend Each Other

In *World of Warcraft*, you have to join up with others to have a chance at challenging tough bosses. Together, everyone combines skills and becomes far more powerful as a group than each individual could hope to be alone. This is how your group of real-life game-playing friends should operate. When everyone works to protect privacy and stay safe, the whole group benefits.

You are closely connected to your friends in the gaming world, just as in real life. You play together, you know each others' gamertags, and you know a lot of real-world information about each other. You probably play on each others' computers and consoles from time to time. Because

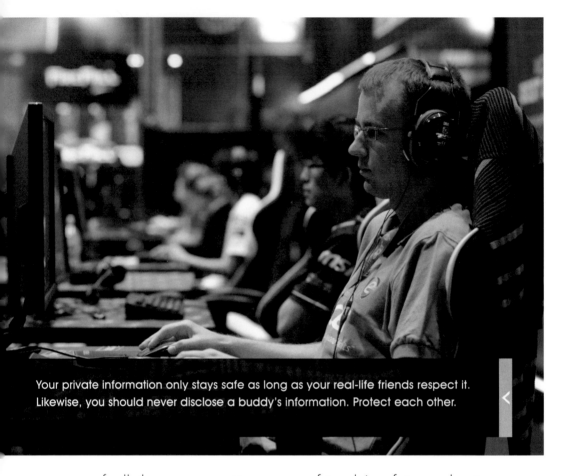

Your private information only stays safe as long as your real-life friends respect it. Likewise, you should never disclose a buddy's information. Protect each other.

of all these connections, your friends' safety and privacy practices affect *your* safety and privacy. This isn't a cause for alarm or reason to be scared, but more of a call to arms: protect your friends' privacy as if it were your own, and ask them to do the same for you.

Guarding your privacy along with a friend can be even more fun than doing so alone. Remember, we're *not* talking about password sharing here! Friends who are in the privacy loop should already know to respect the secrecy of other friends' passwords. Making up anonymous usernames

> PEER PRESSURE AND
> ONLINE GAMING

Peer pressure to do things you don't feel comfortable with can be a problem in groups of friends who enjoy gaming online. Sometimes peer pressure occurs in-game, with friends egging one another to grief and harass others. This isn't acceptable, and it's just as important to resist this kind of influence in-game as it is in real life. Often, you may need to make a stand against nasty behavior before the gameplay even begins.

Many popular online multiplayer games are M-rated, meant for players age seventeen and up. These games often feature violent or lewd content, and they tend to have the worst problems with bad gamer behavior during online play. It's very easy to end up in deep water while playing one of these titles online, drawing taunts and harassment from foul-mouthed, mean-spirited players. Lots of young people want to play these games because they seem "cool"; they seem like the type of games older people would want to play. For some kids, it seems like these games come with a license for rudeness and bad behavior. They don't want to play because of the game itself but because it makes them feel powerful to use foul language and be mean to other gamers.

Don't wallow in a cesspit of profanity, sexism, racism, and homophobia. You shouldn't waste time playing something if the only appeal stems from peer pressure. It's not cowardly to refuse to play a game if you're uncomfortable with the in-game atmosphere. In fact, it takes more courage to stand up and say no than it does to follow along and play something inappropriate just because your friends say it's cool. Encourage your friends to play something else. Choose another game that entertains you through the challenge and joy of its gameplay, rather than the allure of acting cruel.

and avatars with friends, on the other hand, can be a blast, and even result in unparalleled creativity. Your friends can be trusted to know your secret gaming identity. Joining together to play on protected servers, or playing in groups or guilds of friends in games that allow teamwork, can help keep everyone safer. Rather than trying to meet new friends while playing online, ask new people you meet in real life if they play. You might make a new friend and get a new teammate (or opponent, depending on the game) at the same time.

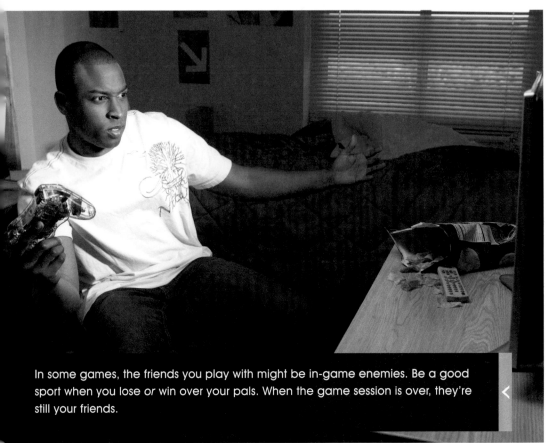

In some games, the friends you play with might be in-game enemies. Be a good sport when you lose *or* win over your pals. When the game session is over, they're still your friends.

Friends have each others' backs in tough gaming situations. If someone griefs or bullies you, your friends should be there to support you. This does *not* mean they should seek in-game retaliation against your harasser. They should be there to offer reasonable verbal or text-based support, and if that doesn't work, to offer moral support and individually report the bad behavior of your antagonist. Likewise, if you witness someone hassle your friend in a game, don't try to grief the person back or yell at him or her out of revenge. Seeking in-game vigilante justice is rarely ever satisfying; it often merely escalates the situation and sets a griefer's sights on multiple members of a friend group. Do what you should do for *anyone* you see being treated unfairly in-game: Ask the bully to stop, and if he or she doesn't, report the actions to your gaming service provider. If an entire group of friends sees a griefer in action and each takes time to report the unacceptable behavior, there's a far greater chance that a game service representative will take action against the bully than if the victim alone reported the harassment. Take a stand as a group to halt antisocial, unsportsmanlike behavior, and report bullies and griefers through the proper channels. Good stewardship benefits everyone who plays the game.

On the other side of the situation, don't let your friends get away with bullying others. If you witness a friend acting out or unfairly targeting another player in-game, take a stand against it. Griefing isn't cool. Let your friends know that you don't consider it acceptable.

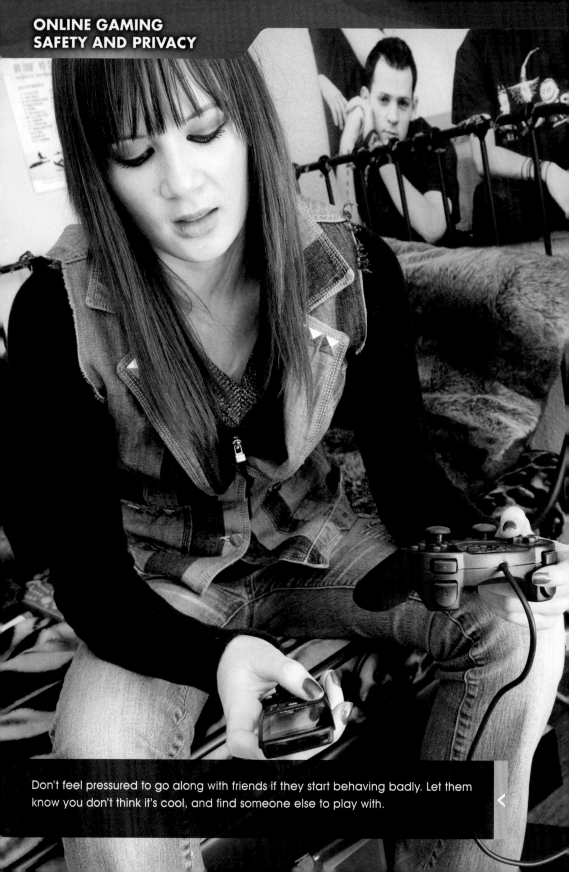

Don't feel pressured to go along with friends if they start behaving badly. Let them know you don't think it's cool, and find someone else to play with.

When a Friend Is in Trouble

You know to watch your own accounts for any signs of strange activity that may indicate you've been hacked. What if it's not you, but your friend who notices an odd purchase on his or her PlayStation Network account? If it seems like your friend may be dealing with a serious problem, don't blow it off. Tell your friend why you think something's wrong, and you should both tell an adult. Don't ignore a warning sign just because your friend seems unconcerned.

This also applies to social issues in online gaming. Does one of your friends behave badly online, continuing to grief others even after you've asked for the behavior to stop? Tell an adult. It might not seem like the cool thing to do, but as other gamers who are fed up with griefing would tell you, it is definitely the best course of action. Don't stand by idly while a friend hurts others and endangers his or her own gaming account by behaving badly.

If a friend develops an inappropriate relationship while playing online, go straight to an adult. When a pal is spending a lot of time talking to a stranger online, it's cause for concern, particularly if he or she begins to act secretively or defensively about his or her gaming communication. Don't let a friend be duped by a shady online character. Let an adult know about the situation, and offer your friend real-life support and loyalty to show you care.

GLOSSARY

avatar A pictorial or three-dimensional representation of a gaming service user.

block An action undertaken by a gaming service user to prevent another user from seeing or contacting the first user.

ESRB The Entertainment Software Rating Board, which assigns age and content ratings for video games and mobile apps, enforces advertising and marketing guidelines for the video game industry, and helps companies implement responsible online privacy practices.

gamer A person who plays computer or video games.

gamertag Xbox Live's term for a user's online identity.

gaming service A network such as the Nintendo Wi-Fi Network, PlayStation Network, or Xbox Live that allows users to play online games and download digital media.

griefing The act of purposefully irritating and harassing other players in an online multiplayer video game. A person who participates in griefing is known as a griefer.

hack To gain access to or alter an electronic file, program, or network illicitly.

in-game Describing conversation or actions undertaken by a player in the virtual world of a video game, rather than in normal life.

jacker Informal slang for a computer or game account hijacker who takes control of an account and forces its rightful owner out.

MMORPG Abbreviation for massively multiplayer online role-playing game, such as *World of Warcraft*.

phishing A type of online scam in which a hacker tricks someone into revealing personal information that the hacker may then use illicitly.

platform The console or gaming service someone uses to play an online game, such as Xbox 360 or Xbox Live.

PSN Abbreviation for PlayStation Network, Sony's online gaming service.

real-world Describing something belonging to the world outside of a gaming reality; also called real-life.

report An action undertaken to inform a game or gaming service about undesirable behavior on the part of a user.

social engineering A type of phishing attack in which a hacker gains information about a person by impersonating the victim in communication with a company's customer service representative.

user agreement Legal contract between a software application author or publisher and the end user of that application to comply with all restrictions stated in said document.

username A pseudonym used to identify a player in an online game.

Canadian Centre for Child Protection, Inc.
615 Academy Road
Winnipeg, MB, R3N 0E7
Canada
Web site: https://www.cybertip.ca
Operated by the Canadian Centre for Child Protection,
Cybertip!ca works to protect children from online
sexual exploitation by receiving and reporting tips
about illegal activity and providing educational
resources to help families stay safe online.

Childnet International
Studio 14 Brockley Cross Business Centre
96 Endwell Road
London SE4 2PD
Web site: http://www.childnet.com
Childnet International partners with organizations around
the world to promote quality content for young people,
raise awareness and provide advice about Internet
safety, and initiate policy changes to protect children
from online exploitation.

Federal Bureau of Investigation
Cyber Division
Innocent Images National Initiative

11700 Beltsville Drive
Calverton, MD 20705
Web site: http://www.fbi.gov/stats-services/publica-
    tions/parent-guide/parent-guide
A Parent's Guide to Internet Safety provides detailed
    information to help parents understand the complexities
    of online child exploitation and protect their children
    from fear and victimization.

NetSmartzKids
Charles B. Wang International
Children's Building
699 Prince Street
Alexandria, VA 22314-3175
Web site: http://www.netsmartzkids.org
NetSmartz Workshop is an interactive educational pro-
    gram designed to help children ages five to seventeen
    stay safe on- and offline, providing resources such as
    videos, games, activity cards, and presentations to
    entertain and educate.

NSTeens
Charles B. Wang International
Children's Building
699 Prince Street

Alexandria, VA 22314-3175

Web site: http://www.nsteens.org

NSTeens' free resources, which include animated educational videos and real-life stories about teens' online experiences, empower tweens and teens to make safer choices online.

Smithsonian American Art Museum

P.O. Box 37012

SI Building, Room 153, MRC 010

Washington, DC 20013-7012

Web site: http://americanart.si.edu/exhibitions/ archive/2012/games/

Focusing on the interplay between graphics, technology, and storytelling, "The Art of Video Games" is one of the first exhibitions to explore the forty-year evolution of video games as an artistic medium.

Web Sites

Due to the changing nature of Internet links, Rosen Publishing has developed an online list of Web sites related to the subject of this book. This site is updated regularly. Please use this link to access the list:

http://www.rosenlinks.com/21C/Game

Cline, Ernest. *Ready Player One: A Novel.* New York, NY: Crown Publishers, 2011.

Day-Macleod, Deirdre. *Viruses and Spam.* New York, NY: Rosen Publishing Group, 2008.

Gilsdorg, Ethan. *Fantasy Freaks and Gaming Geeks: An Epic Quest for Reality Among Role Players, Online Gamers, and Other Dwellers of Imaginary Realms.* Guilford, CT: Lyons Press, 2009.

Gregson, Susan Regan. *Cyber Literacy: Evaluating the Reliability of Data.* New York, NY: Rosen Publishing Group, 2008.

Harbour, Jonathan S. *Video Game Programming for Kids.* Independence, KY: Course Technology PTR, 2012.

Jakubiak, David J. *A Smart Kid's Guide to Avoiding Online Predators.* New York, NY: Rosen Publishing Group, 2010.

Jakubiak, David J. *A Smart Kid's Guide to Internet Privacy.* New York, NY: Rosen Publishing Group, 2010.

Jakubiak, David J. *A Smart Kid's Guide to Online Bullying.* New York, NY: Rosen Publishing Group, 2010.

Jakubiak, David J. *A Smart Kid's Guide to Playing Online Games.* New York, NY: Rosen Publishing Group, 2010.

Jenisch, Josh. *The Art of the Video Game.* Philadelphia, PA: Quirk Books, 2008.

Jones, David Kent. *Online Teen Dangers: The Five Greatest Internet Dangers Teenagers Face and What You Can Do to Protect Them.* Seattle, WA: CreateSpace, 2008.

Marcovitz, Hal. *Online Gaming and Entertainment* (Issues in the Digital Age). San Diego, CA: ReferencePoint Press, 2011.

Melissinos, Christopher, and Patrick O'Rourke. *The Art of Video Games: From Pac-Man to Mass Effect.* New York, NY: Welcome Books, 2012.

Orr, Tamra B. *Privacy and Hacking.* New York, NY: Rosen Publishing Group, 2008.

Spivet, Bonnie. *Avoiding Predators Online.* New York, NY: Rosen Publishing Group, 2012.

Spivet, Bonnie. *Playing Games Online.* New York, NY: Rosen Publishing Group, 2012.

Spivet, Bonnie. *Protecting Your Privacy Online.* New York, NY: Rosen Publishing Group, 2012.

Spivet, Bonnie. *Stopping Cyberbullying.* New York, NY: Rosen Publishing Group, 2012.

Willard, Nancy E. *Cyber-Safe Kids, Cyber-Savvy Teens: Helping Young People Learn to Use the Internet Safely and Responsibly.* San Francisco, CA: Jossey-Bass, 2007.

Williams, J. Patrick. *Gaming as Culture: Essays on Reality, Identity and Experience in Fantasy Games.* Jefferson, NC: McFarland, 2006.

Arendt, Susan. "Study: Online Gaming Good for Teens." *Wired*. Retrieved October 7, 2012 (http://www .wired.com/gamelife/2007/07/study-online-ga).

Castillo, Michelle. "Video Games: When Girl Gamers Go Pro." Time Entertainment. Retrieved October 7, 2012 (http://www.time.com/time/arts/article /0,8599,2024773,00.html).

Dolak, Abbey, Jennifer Dolak, and Kevin Dolak. "Parents Relieved to Have 13-Year-Old Daughter Home After 900-Mile Trip to See 12-Year-Old Boy." *ABC News*. Retrieved October 7, 2012 (http://abcnews.go.com /US/parents-relieved-13-year-daughter-home-900 -mile/story?id=17191315#.UHlXPGjyZOg).

Entertainment Software Association. "2012 Sales, Demographic and Usage Data: Essential Facts About the Computer and Video Game Industry." Retrieved November 2012 (http://www.theesa.com/facts /pdfs/ESA_EF_2012.pdf).

Entertainment Software Ratings Board. "ESRB Rating & Content Descriptor Guide." Retrieved October 7, 2012 (http://www.esrb.org/ratings/ratings_guide.jsp).

Hayes, Eric. "Playing It Safe: Avoiding Online Gaming Risks." US-CERT. Retrieved October 7, 2012 (http:// www.us-cert.gov/reading_room/gaming.pdf).

Hayes, Rob. "Online Video Games May Expose Kids to Violent Language, Experts Warn." *ABC News*.

Retrieved October 7, 2012 (http://abclocal.go.com
/kabc/story?section=news/consumer&id=8596874).

Jenkins, Henry. "Reality Bytes: Eight Myths About Video
Games Debunked." PBS. Retrieved October 7, 2012
(http://www.pbs.org/kcts/videogamerevolution
/impact/myths.html).

McGonigal, Jane. *Reality Is Broken: Why Games Make
Us Better and How They Can Change the World.*
New York, NY: Penguin Books, 2011.

Microsoft Safety & Security Center. "Online Gaming:
Help Kids Play It Safe." Retrieved October 7, 2012
(http://www.microsoft.com/security/family-safety
/gaming-about.aspx).

Pew Internet & American Life Project. "Teens, Video
Games and Civics." Pew Research Center
Publications. Retrieved October 7, 2012 (http://
pewresearch.org/pubs/953).

Poisso, Lisa. "A Parent's Guide to World of Warcraft for
Kids." WoW Insider. Retrieved October 7, 2012
(http://wow.joystiq.com/2011/04/27/a-parents
-guide-to-world-of-warcraft-for-kids).

Schreier, Jason. "Confessions of a Teenage Xbox Hacker."
Kotaku. Retrieved October 7, 2012 (http://kotaku.
com/5948617/confessions-of-a-teenage-xbox
-hacker?popular=true).

Schreier, Jason. "PlayStation Network Hack Leaves Credit
Card Info at Risk." Wired. Retrieved October 7, 2012

(http://www.wired.com/gamelife/2011/04
/playstation-network-hacked).

Science Daily. "Study Examines Video Game Play Among
Adolescents." Retrieved October 7, 2012 (http://
www.sciencedaily.com/releases/2007/07/07070
2161141.htm).

Smith, Leonie. "Should Your Children Play Online
Games?" The Cyber Safety Lady. Retrieved October
7, 2012 (http://thecybersafetylady.com.au/2012
/02/should-your-children-play-online-games).

STOP Cyberbullying. "Direct Attacks: Cyberbullying by
Proxy." Retrieved October 7, 2012 (http://www
.stopcyberbullying.org/how_it_works/direct
_attacks.html).

Taylor, Susan. "Microsoft: A Tale of Bad Customer
Service." Hacked on Xbox. Retrieved October 7,
2012 (http://www.hackedonxbox.com/microsoft).

Taylor, Susan. "Sean B's Very Happy Ending." Hacked
on Xbox. Retrieved October 7, 2012 (http://www
.hackedonxbox.com/sean-bs-very-happy-ending).

Thompson, Mike. "Woman Seduces Teen She Met on
Xbox Live, Gets Busted." Escapist Magazine. Retrieved
October 7, 2012 (http://www.escapistmagazine
.com/news/view/106808-Woman-Seduces
-Teen-She-Met-on-Xbox-Live-Gets-Busted).

INDEX

About the Author

Jennifer Culp is a writer, artist, and lifelong video game lover. She writes about women and video games for a number of online publications.

Photo Credits

Cover (figure) © Monkey Business Images/Shutterstock .com; cover (background), p. 27 Bloomberg/Getty Images; p. 4 Kevork Djansezian/Getty Images; p. 7 Stephen Brasher/Invision for Xbox/AP Images; p. 9 Hemera/Thinkstock; pp. 12, 16, 18 © AP Images; p. 22 OJO Images/Getty Images; p. 29 © Jan Knoff/ DPA/ZUMA Press; p. 34 Tetra Images/Getty Images; p. 38 Monkey Business Images/The Agency Collection/ Getty Images; p. 40 Richard Clark/Photolibrary/Getty Images; p. 43 iStockphoto/Thinkstock; p. 46 Juergen Schwarz/Getty Images; p. 48 James Woodson/Digital Vision/Thinkstock; p. 50 Ingram Publishing/Thinkstock.

Designer: Brian Garvey; Editor: Bethany Bryan; Photo Researcher: Amy Feinberg